Traditional Vegetarian Meatless Recipes

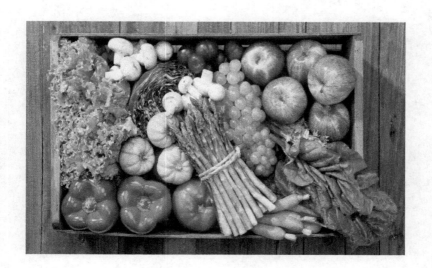

2 books in 1: Improve your skills right now and skip the busy kitchen with this collection of quick recipe, selected to help you lose weight and build a completely meatless meal plan.

Joe Madison

Welcome

To the vegetarian world!

A worldwide community, focused on health and sustainability.

Have you ever desired to live a light and healthy life?

This book is going to introduce you to a genuine and **natural way of living.**

Even if you don't fully commit to the vegetarian lifestyle, adding few vegetarian meals into your diet can make a **notable difference**.

In this book, we'll go through many simple recipes to get you started with a vegetarian diet and to give you a quick **and natural boost.**

With this book, you will be deliciated by our selection of dishes, thought to give you:

Super fast recipes

From raw to cooked in the shorter time and with the maximum efficiency. In this book, you'll find many recipes to surprise your guests... and yourself first.

Boost your health

By introducing these recipes in your life, you'll see your mind and body wellness increase quickly.

Mediterranean diet

Learn more recipes ideated in the land of the wellness, to live a longer and tastier life.

New approach to the food

Your ingredients choice will expand and you'll improve your cooking knowledge.

Table of contents Book 1:

Vegetarian Recipes from the Mediterranean Vol. 1

Table of Contents Book 2:
Vegetarian Recipes from the Mediterranean Vol. 2

Vegetarian Recipes

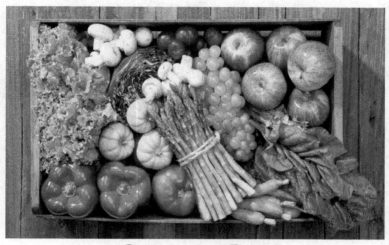

from the
Mediterranean

Vol. 1

This tasteful cookbook will introduce you into a sustainable world of whole-foods, plant-based and lifelong meals. Improve your skills right now with this low-budget, quick and easy cookbook and its 365 days amazing vegs!

JoeMadison

Roasted Tomatoes

Serves 4 pax

Ingredients

- 1/4 teaspoon oregano
- 3/4 cup extra-virgin olive oil
- 3 pounds tomatoes
- 1 teaspoon salt
- 2 garlic cloves
- 1 teaspoon pepper

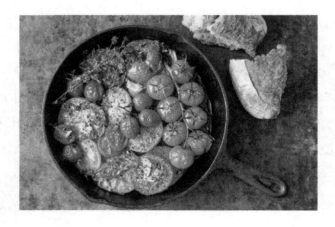

Procedure

1. Place the oven rack in the center of the oven and pre-heat your oven to 425 degrees.
2. Line rimmed baking sheet with aluminium foil. Arrange tomatoes in a uniform layer in readied sheet, with larger slices around edge and smaller slices in center.
3. Place garlic cloves on tomatoes. Sprinkle with oregano and 1/4 teaspoon salt and season with pepper to taste.
4. Sprinkle oil evenly over tomatoes.
5. Bake for 30 minutes, rotating sheet halfway through baking. Remove sheet from oven. Reduce oven temperature to 300 degrees and prop open door with wooden spoon to cool oven.
6. Using thin spatula, flip tomatoes. Return tomatoes to oven, close oven door, and carry on cooking until spotty brown, skins are blistered, and tomatoes have collapsed to 1/4 to 1/2 inch thick, 1 to 2 hours.
7. Remove from oven and allow to cool completely, approximately half an hour. Discard garlic and move tomatoes and oil to airtight container.

Applesauce

Serves 5 cups

Ingredients

- 1/4 cup water
- 1 teaspoon cinnamon
- 4 pounds apples
- 1 teaspoon vanilla extract
- 2 tablespoons lemon juice

Procedure

1. Add apples and water to the Termoblender.
2. Cover and seal lid. Set to manual for 5 minutes.
3. When cooking time ends, quick release pressure and let cool.
4. Add apples, cinnamon, lemon juice, and vanilla to a blender or food processor and blend until smooth.
5. Refrigerate for up to 4 days.
6. Serve.

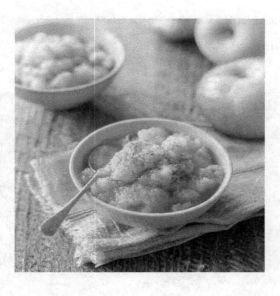

Grilled Radicchio

Serves 5 pax

Ingredients

- 1 garlic clove
- 2 heads radicchio
- 1 teaspoon pepper
- 1 teaspoon rosemary
- 3 tablespoons extra-virgin olive oil
- 1 teaspoon salt

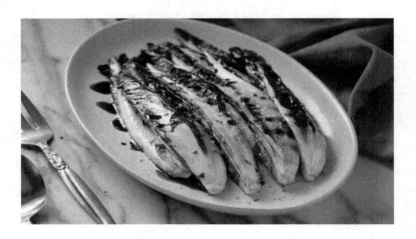

Procedure

1. Microwave oil, garlic, and rosemary in a container until bubbling, approximately one minute. Let mixture steep for about sixty seconds.
2. Brush radicchio with 1/4 cup oil mixture and sprinkle with salt and pepper.
3. With a Charcoal Grill, open bottom vent fully. Light large chimney starter half filled with charcoal briquettes (3 quarts). When top coals are partially covered with ash, pour uniformly over grill. Set cooking grate in place, cover, and open lid vent fully. Heat grill until hot, approximately five minutes.
4. Turn all burners to high, cover, and heat grill until hot, about fifteen minutes. Turn all burners to medium.
5. Clean and oil cooking grate. Place radicchio on grill. Cook (covered if using gas), flipping as required, until radicchio becomes tender and mildly charred, 3 to 5 minutes. Move to serving platter and drizzle with remaining oil mixture. Serve.

Cauliflower Cake

Serves 4 pax

Ingredients

- 1 egg
- 1 teaspoon lemon zest
- 1/4 cup all-purpose flour
- 1/4 cup extra-virgin olive oil
- 1/2 teaspoon ginger
- 1 cauliflower
- 1/4 teaspoon pepper
- 1 teaspoon salt
- 1 teaspoon turmeric
- 4 ounces goat cheese
- 3 garlic cloves
- 2 scallions
- 1 teaspoon coriander

Procedure

1. Place the oven rack in the center of the oven and pre-heat your oven to 450 degrees.
2. Toss cauliflower with 1 tablespoon oil, turmeric, coriander, salt, ginger, and pepper. Move to aluminium foil–lined rimmed baking sheet and spread into one layer.
3. Roast until cauliflower is thoroughly browned and tender, about 25 minutes.
4. Allow it to cool slightly, then move to big container.
5. Line clean rimmed baking sheet with parchment paper. Mash cauliflower coarsely with potato masher.
6. Mix in goat cheese, scallions, egg, garlic, and lemon zest until thoroughly mixed. Sprinkle flour over cauliflower mixture and stir to incorporate.
7. Using wet hands, divide mixture into 4 equal portions, pack gently into 3/4-inch-thick cakes, and place on readied sheet. Refrigerate cakes until chilled and firm, approximately half an hour.

8. Line large plate using paper towels. Heat remaining 3 tablespoons oil in 12-inch non-stick frying pan on moderate heat until it starts to shimmer.

9. Gently lay cakes in frying pan and cook until deep golden brown and crisp, 5 to 7 minutes each side.

10. Drain cakes briefly on prepared plate.

11. Serve with lemon wedges.

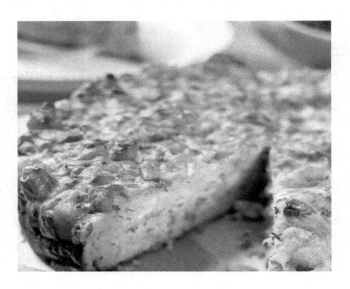

Fava Beans

Serves 6 pax

Ingredients

- 3 pounds asparagus
- 2 pounds fava beans
- 2 pounds peas
- 2 tablespoons basil
- 2 teaspoons lemon zest
- 1 tablespoon mint
- 1 cup vegetable broth
- 1 leek
- 1 tablespoon extra-virgin olive oil
- 1 teaspoon baking soda
- 2 garlic cloves
- 2 artichokes
- 2 teaspoons salt
- 2 teaspoons pepper

Procedure

1. Cut 1 lemon in half, squeeze halves into container filled with 2 quarts water, then put in spent halves.
2. Working with 1 artichoke at a time, trim stem to about 3/4 inch and cut off top quarter of artichoke.
3. Break off bottom 3 or 4 rows of tough outer leaves by pulling them downward. Use a paring knife to trim outer layer of stem and base, removing any dark green parts. Cut artichoke into quarters and submerge in lemon water.
4. Bring 2 cups water and baking soda to boil in small saucepan. Put in beans and cook until edges begin to darken, 1 to 2 minutes. Drain and wash thoroughly with cold water.
5. Heat oil in 12-inch frying pan on moderate heat until it starts to shimmer. Put in leek, 1 tablespoon water, and 1 teaspoon salt and cook till they become tender, approximately three minutes.
6. Mix in garlic and cook until aromatic, approximately half a minute.

7. Take artichokes out of lemon water, shaking off excess water, and put into skillet. Mix in broth and bring to simmer.
8. Decrease heat to moderate to low, cover, and cook until artichokes are almost tender, six to eight minutes.
9. Mix in asparagus and peas, cover, and cook until crisp-tender, 5 to 7 minutes.
10. Mix in beans and cook until heated through and artichokes are fully tender, approximately two minutes.
11. Remove from the heat, mix in basil, mint, and lemon zest. Sprinkle with salt and pepper to taste and drizzle with extra oil.
12. Serve instantly.

Garlic Braised Kale

Serves 8 pax

Ingredients

- 1 onion
- 1 tablespoon lemon juice
- 1/4 teaspoon red pepper flakes
- 1 teaspoon pepper
- 10 garlic cloves
- 2 cups vegetable broth
- 1 cup water
- 4 pounds kale
- 2 tablespoons extra-virgin olive oil
- 1 teaspoon salt

Procedure

1. Heat 3 tablespoons oil in a Dutch oven on moderate heat until it starts to shimmer.
2. Put in onion and cook till they become tender and lightly browned, 5 to 7 minutes. Mix in garlic and pepper flakes and cook until aromatic, approximately one minute. Mix in broth, water, and 1/2 teaspoon salt and bring to simmer.
3. Put in one-third of kale, cover, and cook, stirring intermittently, until wilted, 2 to 4 minutes. Replicate the process with the rest of the kale in 2 batches. Carry on cooking, covered, until kale is tender, 13 to fifteen minutes.
4. Remove lid and increase heat to medium-high. Cook, stirring intermittently, until most liquid has been evaporated and greens begin to sizzle, 10 to 12 minutes. Remove from the heat, mix in remaining 3 tablespoons oil and lemon juice. Sprinkle with salt, pepper, and extra lemon juice to taste. Serve.

Garlic Lemon Potatoes

Serves 5 pax

Ingredients

- 2 pounds Yukon Gold potatoes
- 2 tablespoons parsley
- 2 teaspoons lemon zest
- 2 tablespoons lemon juice
- 2 tablespoons extra-virgin olive oil
- 1 teaspoon salt
- 1 teaspoon pepper
- 2 tablespoons oregano
- 2 garlic cloves

Procedure

1. Heat 2 tablespoons oil in 12-inch non-stick frying pan on moderate to high heat until it starts to shimmer.

2. Put in potatoes cut side down in one layer and cook until golden brown on first side (frying pan should sizzle but not smoke), about 6 minutes.

3. Using tongs, flip potatoes onto second cut side and cook until golden brown, approximately five minutes.

4. Decrease heat to moderate to low, cover, and cook until potatoes are tender, 8 to 12 minutes.

5. In the meantime, beat remaining 1 tablespoon oil, oregano, garlic, lemon zest and juice, 1/2 teaspoon salt, and 1/2 teaspoon pepper together in a small-sized container.

6. When potatoes are tender, gently mix in garlic mixture and cook, uncovered, until aromatic, approximately two minutes. Remove from the heat, gently mix in parsley and sprinkle with salt and pepper to taste.

Broccoli Rabe

Serves 4 pax

Ingredients

- 1/4 teaspoon red pepper flakes
- 2 garlic cloves
- 1 teaspoon salt
- 14 ounces broccoli rabe
- 2 tablespoons extra-virgin olive oil
- 1 teaspoon pepper

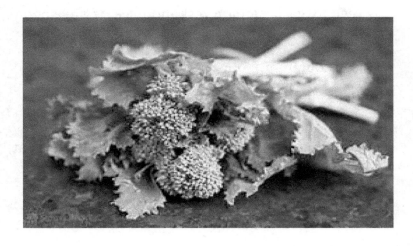

Procedure

1. Bring 3 quarts water to boil in a big saucepan. Fill big container halfway with ice and water.
2. Put in broccoli rabe and 2 teaspoons salt to boiling water and cook until wilted and tender, about 21/2 minutes.
3. Drain broccoli rabe, then move to ice water and allow to sit until chilled. Drain again and thoroughly pat dry.
4. Cook oil, garlic, and pepper flakes in 10-inch frying pan on moderate heat, stirring frequently, until garlic begins to sizzle, approximately two minutes.
5. Increase heat to medium-high, put in broccoli rabe, and cook, stirring to coat with oil, until heated through, approximately one minute.
6. Sprinkle with salt and pepper to taste and serve.

Grilled Zucchini

Serves 4 pax

Ingredients

- 1/4 teaspoon Dijon mustard
- 1 teaspoon lemon zest
- 1 tablespoon lemon juice
- 6 tablespoons extra-virgin olive oil
- 1 teaspoon salt
- 1 garlic clove
- 1 tablespoon basil
- 1 teaspoon pepper
- 1 onion
- 2 pounds zucchini

Procedure

1. Thread onion rounds from side to side onto two 12-inch metal skewers.
2. Brush onion and zucchini with 1/4 cup oil, drizzle with 1 teaspoon salt, and season with pepper.
3. Beat remaining 2 tablespoons oil, lemon zest and juice, garlic, mustard, and 1/4 teaspoon salt together in a container; set aside for serving.
4. Open bottom vent fully. Light large chimney starter half filled with charcoal briquettes (3 quarts). When top coals are partially covered with ash, pour uniformly over grill. Set cooking grate in place, cover, and open lid vent fully. Heat grill until hot, approximately five minutes.
5. Clean and oil cooking grate. Place vegetables cut side down on grill. Cook, turning as required, until soft and caramelized, 18 to 22 minutes.
6. Move vegetables to serving platter as they finish cooking. Remove skewers from onion and discard any charred outer rings. Beat dressing to recombine, then drizzle over vegetables.

Marinated Aubergine

Serves 5 pax

Ingredients

- 1/2 teaspoon oregano
- 1 garlic clove
- 2 teaspoons red wine vinegar
- 2 teaspoons salt
- 1 tablespoon capers
- 11/2 pounds eggplant
- 2 tablespoons mint
- 2 teaspoons pepper
- 1/4 cup extra-virgin olive oil
- 1/2 teaspoon lemon zest

Procedure

1. Lay out eggplant on paper towel–lined baking sheet, drizzle both sides with 1/2 teaspoon salt, and allow to sit for 30 minutes.
2. Place oven rack 4 inches from broiler element and heat broiler. Comprehensively pat eggplant dry using paper towels, arrange on aluminium foil–lined rimmed baking sheet in one layer, and lightly brush both sides with 1 tablespoon oil.
3. Broil eggplant until mahogany brown and mildly charred, six to eight minutes each side.
4. Beat remaining 3 tablespoons oil, vinegar, capers, garlic, lemon zest, oregano, and 1/4 teaspoon pepper together in a big container.
5. Put in eggplant and mint and gently toss to combine. Let eggplant cool to room temperature, about 1 hour.
6. Season with pepper to taste and serve.

Stewed Zucchini

Serves 8 pax

Ingredients

- 1 teaspoon oregano
- 5 zucchini
- 1 teaspoon salt
- 2 tablespoons kalamata olives
- 2 tablespoons mint
- 2 garlic cloves
- 1/4 teaspoon red pepper flakes
- 28 ounces tomatoes
- 1 onion
- 2 tablespoons extra-virgin olive oil
- 1 teaspoon pepper

Procedure

1. Place oven rack to lower-middle position and pre-heat your oven to 325 degrees. Process tomatoes and their juice using a food processor until smoothened thoroughly, approximately one minute. Set aside.

2. Heat 2 teaspoons oil in a Dutch oven on moderate to high heat until just smoking. Brown one-third of zucchini, approximately three minutes each side; move to a container.

3. Repeat with 4 teaspoons oil and remaining zucchini in 2 batches.

4. Put in remaining 1 tablespoon oil, onion, and 3/4 teaspoon salt to now-empty pot and cook, stirring intermittently, over moderate to low heat until onion is very soft and golden brown, 9 to 11 minutes.

5. Mix in garlic, oregano, and pepper flakes and cook until aromatic, approximately half a minute.

6. Mix in olives and tomatoes, bring to simmer, and cook, stirring intermittently, until sauce has thickened, approximately half an hour.
7. Mix in zucchini and any accumulated juice, cover, and move pot to oven.
8. Bake until zucchini is very tender, 30 to 40 minutes.
9. Mix in mint and adjust sauce consistency with hot water as required.
10. Sprinkle with salt and pepper to taste.
11. Serve.

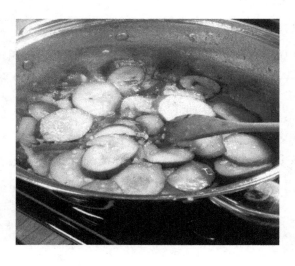

Grilled Aubergine

Ingredients

- 1/8 teaspoon red pepper flakes
- 2 tablespoons extra-virgin olive oil
- 1 teaspoon salt
- 1/2 cup yogurt
- 1 teaspoon lemon zest
- 2 teaspoons lemon juice
- 2 garlic cloves
- 1 teaspoon pepper
- 1 teaspoon cumin
- 3 pounds eggplant
- 2 tablespoons mint

Procedure

1. Mix oil, garlic, and pepper flakes in a container. Microwave until garlic is golden brown and crisp, approximately two minutes.

2. Strain garlic oil through fine-mesh strainer into small-sized container. Reserve garlic oil and garlic separately.

3. Beat 1 tablespoon garlic oil, yogurt, mint, lemon zest and juice, cumin, and 1/4 teaspoon salt together in different container. Set aside for serving.

4. Open bottom vent fully. Light large chimney starter filled with charcoal briquettes (6 quarts).

5. When top coals are partially covered with ash, pour uniformly over grill.

6. Set cooking grate in place, cover, and open lid vent fully. Heat grill until hot, approximately five minutes.

7. Turn all burners to high, cover, and heat grill until hot, about fifteen minutes. Turn all burners to medium-high.

8. Clean and oil cooking grate. Brush eggplant with remaining garlic oil and sprinkle with salt and pepper.

9. Place half of eggplant on grill and cook (covered if using gas) until browned and tender, about 4 minutes each side. Move to serving platter.

10. Replicate the process with the rest of the eggplant. Move to platter.

11. Sprinkle yogurt sauce over eggplant and drizzle with garlic.

12. Serve.

Lemon Artichokes

Serves 4 pax

Ingredients

- 2 teaspoons parsley
- 9 tablespoons extra-virgin olive oil
- 2 teaspoons salt
- 3 lemons
- 5 artichokes
- 2 teaspoons pepper
- 1/2 teaspoon Dijon mustard
- 1/2 teaspoon garlic

Procedure

1. Place oven rack to lower-middle position and pre-heat your oven to 475 degrees. Cut 1 lemon in half, squeeze halves into container filled with 2 quarts water, then put in spent halves.
2. Working with 1 artichoke at a time, trim stem to about 3/4 inch and cut off top quarter of artichoke. Break off bottom 3 or 4 rows of tough outer leaves by pulling them downward.
3. Use a paring knife to trim outer layer of stem and base, removing any dark green parts. Cut artichoke in half along the length, then remove fuzzy choke and any tiny inner purple-tinged leaves with the help of a small spoon. Immerse prepped artichokes in lemon water.
4. Coat bottom of 13 by 9-inch baking dish with 1 tablespoon oil. Take artichokes out of lemon water and shake off water, leaving some water still remaining on leaves.

5. Toss artichokes with 2 tablespoons oil, 3/4 teaspoon salt, and pinch pepper. Gently rub oil and

6. seasonings between leaves. Arrange artichokes cut side down in prepared dish. Trim ends off remaining 2 lemons, halve crosswise, and arrange cut side up next to artichokes.

7. Cover tightly with aluminium foil and roast until cut sides of artichokes begin to brown and bases and leaves are soft when poked with tip of paring knife, about half an hour.

8. Move artichokes to serving platter. Let lemons cool slightly, then squeeze into fine-mesh strainer set over bowl, extracting as much juice and pulp as possible. Press firmly on solids to yield 11/2 tablespoons juice. Beat garlic, mustard, and 1/2 teaspoon salt into juice.

9. Whisking continuously, slowly drizzle in remaining 6 tablespoons oil until completely blended.

10. Beat in parsley and sprinkle with salt and pepper.

11. Serve artichokes with dressing.

Yemen Ratatouille

Serves 5 pax

Ingredients

- 1/4 teaspoon red pepper flakes
- 3 zucchini
- 2 tablespoons basil
- 8 garlic cloves
- 1/3 cup extra-virgin olive oil
- 1 bay leaf
- 1 red bell pepper
- 2 pounds eggplant
- 2 teaspoons herbs de Provence
- 2 onions
- 4 pounds plum tomatoes
- 1 teaspoon salt
- 1 teaspoon pepper
- 1 tablespoon parsley
- 1 tablespoon sherry vinegar

Procedure

1. Place the oven rack in the center of the oven and pre-heat your oven to 400 degrees. Heat 1/3 cup oil in a Dutch oven on moderate to high heat until it starts to shimmer.

2. Put in onions, garlic, 1 teaspoon salt, and 1/4 teaspoon pepper and cook, stirring intermittently, until onions are translucent and starting to soften, about 10 minutes.

3. Put in herbs de Provence, pepper flakes, and bay leaf and cook, stirring often, for about sixty seconds. Mix in eggplant and tomatoes. Sprinkle with 1/2 teaspoon salt and 1/4 teaspoon pepper and stir to combine.

4. Move pot to oven and cook, uncovered, until vegetables are very soft and spotty brown, 40 to 45 minutes.

5. Remove pot from oven and, using potato masher or heavy wooden spoon, smash and stir eggplant mixture until broken down to sauce like consistency.

6. Mix in zucchini, bell peppers, 1/4 teaspoon salt, and 1/4 teaspoon pepper and return to oven.
7. Cook, uncovered, until zucchini and bell peppers are just tender, 20 minutes to half an hour.
8. Remove pot from oven, cover, and allow to sit until zucchini is translucent and easily pierced with tip of paring knife, 10 to fifteen minutes.
9. Using wooden spoon, scrape any browned bits from sides of pot and stir back into ratatouille.
10. Discard bay leaf. Mix in 1 tablespoon basil, parsley, and vinegar. Sprinkle with salt and pepper to taste.
11. Move ratatouille to serving platter, drizzle with remaining 1 tablespoon oil, and drizzle with remaining 1 tablespoon basil.
12. Serve.

Roasted Asparagus

Serves 5 pax

Ingredients

- 1/4 teaspoon pepper
- 2 tablespoons extra-virgin olive oil
- 1/2 teaspoon salt
- 2 pounds asparagus

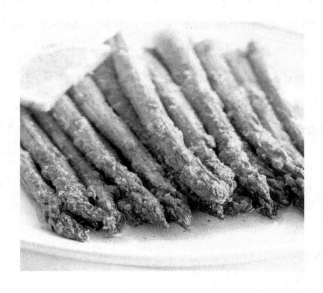

Procedure

1. Place oven rack to lowest position, place rimmed baking sheet on rack, and preheat your oven to 500 degrees.
2. Peel bottom halves of asparagus spears until white flesh is exposed, then toss with 2 tablespoons oil, salt, and pepper.
3. Move asparagus to preheated sheet and spread into one layer. Roast, without moving asparagus, until undersides of spears become browned, tops are bright green, and tip of paring knife inserted at base of largest spear meets little resistance, eight to ten minutes.
4. Move asparagus to serving platter and drizzle with remaining 2 teaspoons oil.
5. Serve.

Carrot Cilantro

Ingredients

- 1/8 teaspoon cinnamon
- 1/4 teaspoon cumin
- 3 tablespoons extra-virgin olive oil
- 2 tablespoons orange juice
- 1 teaspoon salt
- 1/2 teaspoon Aleppo pepper
- 1 tablespoon brown sugar
- 1/4 cup cilantro
- 2 pounds carrots
- 1 teaspoon pepper

Procedure

1. Place the oven rack in the center of the oven and pre-heat your oven to 450 degrees.
2. Beat oil, sugar, 1/2 teaspoon salt, and 1/2 teaspoon pepper together in a big container.
3. Cut carrots in half crosswise, then cut along the length into halves or quarters as required to create uniformly sized pieces.
4. Put in carrots to oil mixture and toss to coat. Move to aluminium foil–lined rimmed baking sheet and spread into one layer.
5. Cover sheet tightly with foil and roast for 12 minutes.
6. Remove foil and continue to roast until carrots are thoroughly browned and tender, 16 to 22 minutes, stirring halfway through roasting.
7. Beat orange juice, Aleppo, cumin, and cinnamon together in a big container.
8. Put in carrots and cilantro and gently toss to combine.
9. Sprinkle with salt and pepper to taste and serve.

Celery Root

Serves 6 pax

Ingredients

- 1/4 cup cilantro
- 1 teaspoon coriander seeds
- 2 tablespoons extra-virgin olive oil
- 1 teaspoon salt
- 1/4 cup plain yogurt
- 1 teaspoon sesame seeds
- 2 celery roots
- 1/4 teaspoon thyme
- 1/4 teaspoon lemon zest
- 1 teaspoon lemon juice
- 1 teaspoon pepper

Procedure

1. Place oven rack on the lowest position and pre-heat your oven to 425 degrees. Toss celery root with oil, 1/2 teaspoon salt, and 1/4 teaspoon pepper and lay out on rimmed baking sheet in one layer.

2. Roast celery root until sides touching sheet toward back of oven are well browned, about half an hour. Rotate sheet and continue to roast until sides touching sheet toward back of oven are well browned, 6 to 10 minutes.

3. Use metal spatula to flip each piece and continue to roast until celery root is very soft and sides touching sheet become browned, 10 to fifteen minutes.

4. Move celery root to serving platter. Beat yogurt, lemon zest and juice, and pinch salt together in a container. In a different container, combine sesame seeds, coriander seeds, thyme, and pinch salt.

5. Sprinkle celery root with yogurt sauce and drizzle with seed mixture and cilantro.

6. Serve.

Roasted Green Beans

Serves 6 pax

Ingredients

- 2 tablespoons pine nuts
- 1 teaspoon salt
- 1 teaspoon Dijon mustard
- 1 teaspoon lemon zest
- 1 tablespoon lemon juice
- 1/4 cup extra-virgin olive oil
- 1/4 cup Pecorino cheese
- 2 pounds green beans
- 2 garlic cloves
- 1 teaspoon pepper
- 3/4 teaspoon sugar
- 2 tablespoons basil

Procedure

1. Place oven rack on the lowest position and pre-heat your oven to 475 degrees. Toss green beans with 1 tablespoon oil, sugar, 1/4 teaspoon salt, and 1/2 teaspoon pepper. Move to rimmed baking sheet and spread into one layer.

2. Cover sheet tightly with aluminium foil and roast for about ten minutes.

3. Remove foil and continue to roast until green beans are spotty brown, about 10 minutes, stirring halfway through roasting.

4. In the meantime, combine garlic, lemon zest, and remaining 3 tablespoons oil in a moderate-sized container and microwave until bubbling, approximately one minute. Let mixture steep for about sixty seconds, then beat in lemon juice, mustard, 1/8 teaspoon salt, and 1/4 teaspoon pepper until combined.

5. Move green beans to a container with dressing, put in basil, and toss to combine. Sprinkle with salt and pepper to taste.

Sautéed Cabbage

Serves 5 pax

Ingredients

- 1/4 cup parsley
- 2 teaspoons lemon juice
- 2 tablespoons extra-virgin olive oil
- 1 teaspoon salt
- 1 green cabbage
- 1 onion
- 1 teaspoon pepper

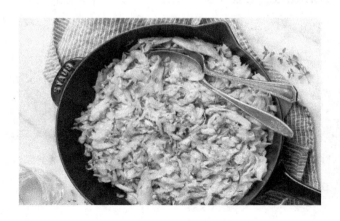

Procedure

1. Place cabbage in a big container and cover with cold water. Allow to sit for about three minutes. Drain well.

2. Heat 1 tablespoon oil in 12-inch non-stick frying pan on moderate to high heat until it starts to shimmer. Put in onion and 1/4 teaspoon salt and cook till they become tender and lightly browned, 5 to 7 minutes; move to a container.

3. Heat residual 1 tablespoon oil in now-empty frying pan on moderate to high heat until it starts to shimmer.

4. Put in cabbage and drizzle with 1/2 teaspoon salt and 1/4 teaspoon pepper. Cover and cook, without stirring, until cabbage is wilted and lightly browned on bottom, approximately three minutes.

5. Stir and continue to cook, uncovered, until cabbage is crisp-tender and lightly browned in places, about 4 minutes, stirring once halfway through cooking.

6. Remove from the heat, mix in onion, parsley, and lemon juice. Serve.

Roasted Mushrooms

Serves 4 pax

Ingredients

- 1 teaspoon lemon juice
- 2 tablespoons extra-virgin olive oil
- 1 teaspoon salt
- 2 pounds cremini mushrooms
- 2 tablespoons parsley
- 2 tablespoons pine nuts
- 1 teaspoon pepper
- 1/2 cup Parmesan cheese
- 1 pound shiitake mushrooms

Procedure

1. Place oven rack on the lowest position and pre-heat your oven to 450 degrees.
2. Dissolve 5 teaspoons salt in 2 quarts room-temperature water in large container. Put in cremini mushrooms and shiitake mushrooms, cover with plate or bowl to submerge, and soak at room temperature for about ten minutes.
3. Drain mushrooms and pat dry using paper towels. Toss mushrooms with 2 tablespoons oil, then spread into one layer in rimmed baking sheet.
4. Roast until liquid from mushrooms has completely evaporated, 35 to 45 minutes.
5. Remove sheet from oven (be careful of escaping steam when opening oven) and, using metal spatula, carefully stir mushrooms.
6. Return to oven and continue to roast until mushrooms are deeply browned, 5 to 10 minutes.
7. Beat residual 1 tablespoon oil and lemon juice together in a big container.
8. Put in mushrooms and toss to coat. Mix in Parmesan, pine nuts, and parsley.

Sautéed Zucchini

Serves 5 pax

Ingredients

- 8 ounces zucchini
- 1 teaspoon salt
- 2 tablespoons parsley
- 3 tablespoons extra-virgin olive oil
- 1 teaspoon pepper
- 1 garlic clove
- 1 teaspoon lemon zest
- 1 tablespoon lemon juice

Procedure

1. Mix garlic and lemon juice in a big container and set aside for minimum 10 minutes. Take a vegetable peeler and use it to shave off 3 ribbons from 1 side of summer squash, then turn squash 90 degrees and shave off 3 more ribbons. Continue to turn and shave ribbons until you reach seeds. Discard core. Replicate the process with the rest of the squash.

2. Beat 2 tablespoons oil, 1/4 teaspoon salt, 1/8 teaspoon pepper, and lemon zest into garlic–lemon juice mixture.

3. Heat remaining 1 teaspoon oil in 12-inch non-stick frying pan on moderate to high heat until just smoking. Put in summer squash and cook, tossing occasionally with tongs, until squash has softened and is translucent, three to five minutes.

4. Move squash to a container with dressing, put in parsley, and gently toss to coat.

5. Sprinkle with salt and pepper to taste.

6. Serve.

Braised Green Beans

Serves 6 pax

Ingredients

- 1/2 teaspoon baking soda
- 14.5 ounces tomatoes
- 1 tablespoon tomato paste
- 2 cups water
- 2 tablespoons extra-virgin olive oil
- 2 tablespoons lemon juice
- 1 teaspoon salt
- 2 pounds green beans
- 3 tablespoons oregano
- 1 onion
- 2 pounds Yukon Gold potatoes
- 2 tablespoons basil
- 2 garlic cloves
- 1 teaspoon pepper

Procedure

1. Place oven rack to lower-middle position and pre-heat your oven to 275 degrees.
2. Heat 3 tablespoons oil in a Dutch oven on moderate heat until it starts to shimmer. Put in onion and cook till they become tender, approximately five minutes.
3. Mix in oregano and garlic and cook until aromatic, approximately half a minute. Mix in water, green beans, potatoes, and baking soda, bring to simmer, and cook, stirring intermittently, for about ten minutes.
4. Mix in tomatoes and their juice, tomato paste, 2 teaspoons salt, and 1/4 teaspoon pepper. Cover, move pot to oven, and cook until sauce is slightly thickened and green beans can be cut easily with side of fork, forty to fifty minutes.
5. Mix in basil and season with salt, pepper, and lemon juice to taste. Move green beans to serving bowl and drizzle with remaining 2 tablespoons oil.
6. Serve.

Sautéed Swiss Chard

Serves 4 pax

Ingredients

- 2 pounds Swiss chard
- 2 teaspoons lemon juice
- 2 garlic cloves
- 2 teaspoons salt
- 3 tablespoons extra-virgin olive oil
- 2 teaspoons pepper

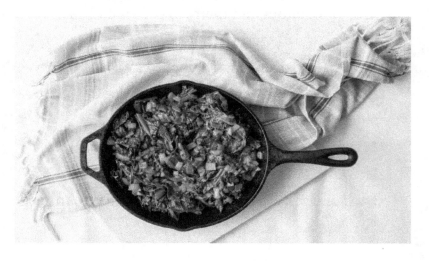

Procedure

1. Heat oil in 12-inch non-stick frying pan on moderate to high heat until it barely starts shimmering. Put in garlic and cook, stirring continuously, until lightly browned, 30 to 60 seconds.
2. Put in chard stems and 1/8 teaspoon salt and cook, stirring intermittently, until spotty brown and crisp-tender, about 6 minutes.
3. Put in two-thirds of chard leaves and cook, tossing with tongs, until just starting to wilt, 30 to 60 seconds.
4. Put in remaining chard leaves and continue to cook, stirring often, until leaves are tender, approximately three minutes.
5. Remove from the heat, mix in lemon juice and sprinkle with salt and pepper to taste.
6. Serve.

Roasted Root Vegetables

Serves 5 pax

Ingredients

- 1 pound Brussels sprouts
- 1 teaspoon rosemary
- 2 teaspoons thyme
- 2 tablespoons extra-virgin olive oil
- 1 teaspoon sugar
- 2 tablespoons capers
- 2 tablespoons parsley
- 2 carrots
- 6 garlic cloves
- 8 shallots
- 2 teaspoons salt
- 1 pound red potatoes
- 1 tablespoon lemon juice

Procedure

1. Place the oven rack in the center of the oven and pre-heat your oven to 450 degrees.
2. Toss Brussels sprouts, potatoes, shallots, and carrots with garlic, 1 tablespoon oil, thyme, rosemary, sugar, 3/4 teaspoon salt, and 1/4 teaspoon pepper.
3. Lay out vegetables into one layer in rimmed baking sheet, arranging Brussels sprouts cut side down in center of sheet.
4. Roast until vegetables are soft and golden brown, 30 to 35 minutes, rotating sheet halfway through roasting.
5. Beat parsley, capers, lemon juice, and remaining 2 tablespoons oil together in a big container.
6. Put in roasted vegetables and toss to combine.
7. Sprinkle with salt and extra lemon juice to taste.
8. Serve.

Zucchini Fritters

Serves 5 pax

Ingredients

- 1/4 cup all-purpose flour
- 2 scallions
- 2 eggs
- 2 lemon wedges
- 2 teaspoons salt
- 2 tablespoons dill
- 2 ounces feta cheese
- 6 tablespoons extra-virgin olive oil
- 1 garlic clove
- 1 pound zucchini
- 2 teaspoons pepper

Procedure

1. Place the oven rack in the center of the oven and pre-heat your oven to 200 degrees. Toss zucchini with 1 teaspoon salt and allow to drain using a fine-mesh strainer for about ten minutes.
2. Wrap zucchini in clean dish towel, squeeze out excess liquid, and move to big container.
3. Mix in feta, scallions, eggs, dill, garlic, and 1/4 teaspoon pepper.
4. Sprinkle flour over mixture and stir to incorporate.
5. Heat 3 tablespoons oil in 12-inch non-stick frying pan on moderate heat until it starts to shimmer.
6. Drop 2-tablespoon-size portions of batter into frying pan and use back of spoon to press batter into 2-inch-wide fritter (you should fit about 6 fritters in frying pan at a time).
7. Fry until golden brown, approximately three minutes each side. Move fritters to paper towel–lined baking sheet and keep warm in oven.
8. Wipe frying pan clean using paper towels and repeat with remaining 3 tablespoons oil and remaining batter.
9. Serve with lemon wedges.

Stuffed Mushrooms

Serves 3 pax

Ingredients

- 1 tsp olive oil
- 1 tsp balsamic vinegar
- 8 oz white mushrooms
- 1 tbsp Parmesan cheese
- 0.25 green pepper
- 0.25 onion
- 1 tbsp mozzarella cheese
- 1 tbsp breadcrumbs

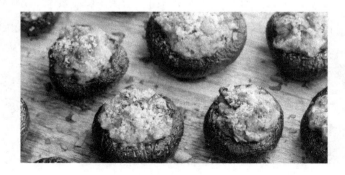

Procedure

1. Take the stems out of the mushrooms and chop them into small pieces. Set aside for now.
2. Marinate the mushroom caps with 1 tsp. olive oil and balsamic vinegar; set aside.
3. Prepare a medium-sized skillet using the medium-temperature setting to heat one teaspoon of oil.
4. Sauté the onion, green pepper, and mushroom stems for three minutes. Cook until completely browned, stirring frequently, about 8-10 minutes.
5. Stir in the breadcrumbs and mozzarella cheese, stirring until the cheese is melted. Remove from heat and mix in the parmesan cheese.
6. Fill each mushroom cap with the mixture, about 1 heaping Tbsp. per cap.
7. Place them in a baking pan coated with nonstick spray and bake at 325°F until the stuffing is crispy on top, about 40 minutes.
8. Serve.

Onion Cornbread

Serves 8 pax

Ingredients

- 2 cups organic cornmeal
- 1/4 cup cilantro
- 1/4 cup coconut oil
- 1 cup maple syrup
- 1/2 cup spelt flour
- 1 teaspoon baking soda
- 1 cup organic corn
- 2 cups almond milk
- 1/2 teaspoon salt
- 1/4 cup green onion
- 1 tablespoon vegan butter
- 5 tablespoons water

Procedure

1. Add 1 cup of water to the Termoblender and grease a 6-7"cake pan. Set aside.
2. In a large bowl, whisk cornmeal, spelt, baking soda and sea salt.
3. Add the green onions, and cilantro.
4. Add the corn kernels and mix gently until well combined.
5. In another bowl, whisk almond milk, coconut oil maple syrup.
6. Pour the wet ingredients into the dry ingredients and gently stir until just combined.
7. Pour the batter into the prepared baking pan and top with a paper towel, then aluminum foil.
8. Put the trivet inside and place the baking pan on top.
9. On manual setting, cook for 25 minutes on high pressure.
10. When it is done, quick release, remove pan, foil and paper towel. Allow to cool and serve.
11. Serve.

Artichoke and Spinach Stuffed Mushrooms

Serves 3 pax

Ingredients

- 1 red onion
- 2 teaspoons salt
- 1 tablespoon garlic
- 1 artichoke
- 2 teaspoons lemon zest
- 1/2 cup breadcrumbs
- 3 Portobello mushrooms
- 2 teaspoons pepper
- 1 pound spinach
- 1 tablespoon olive oil

Procedure

1. On sautèe setting, heat olive oil and add onions and garlic. Sautèe for 4 minutes until onions are soft.
2. Add spinach and cook until wilted.
3. If there is any liquid, drain.
4. Add the artichoke hearts, lemon zest and 1/4 of the breadcrumbs. Add more breadcrumbs if mixture is too wet. Add sea salt and pepper to taste as desired.
5. Remove liner with filling and set aside.
6. Arrange mushrooms on a 6-7" 1/2 inches deep baking pan or foil pan. It is okay if mushrooms overlap because they will cook down.
7. Fill mushrooms with filling. Cover with foil.
8. Add 1 cup of water and place the steamer rack inside the pot. Put the lid on and seal.
9. Set manually for 5 minutes and quick release.
10. Remove pan with oven mitts and remove foil.

Edamame

Serves 6 pax

Ingredients

- 1 tablespoon butter
- 1 clove garlic
- 1 cup vegetable broth
- 1 cup cherry tomatoes
- 2 tablespoons parsley
- 10 ounces edamame beans
- 1 cup corn
- 2 tablespoons basil
- 1 tablespoon balsamic vinegar
- 1 teaspoon salt
- 1 teaspoon extra-virgin olive oil
- 1 cup red onion

Procedure

1. On sautèe mode, heat vegan butter and olive oil together.
2. Cook onion for 5 minutes until soft.
3. Add garlic and cook for 1 minute.
4. Add edamame and cook for 5 minutes.
5. Add the corn and heat through for 1 minute.
6. Add broth and stir to combine the ingredients.
7. Cook on high pressure for 4 minutes.
8. Quick release when done and stir in the tomatoes, parsley, basil and balsamic vinegar.
9. Add sea salt to taste.
10. Serve immediately.

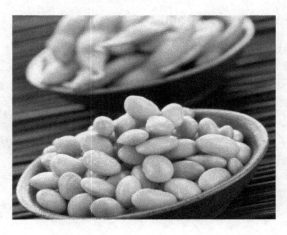

Roasted Squash

Serves 6 pax

Ingredients

- 3 pounds butternut squash
- 2 tablespoons extra-virgin olive oil
- 1 teaspoon salt
- 1 teaspoon honey
- 1/4 cup pistachios
- 1 ounce feta cheese
- 1 tablespoon tahini
- 2 teaspoons lemon juice
- 2 tablespoons mint
- 1 teaspoon pepper

Procedure

1. Place oven rack on the lowest position and pre-heat your oven to 425 degrees.

2. Using sharp vegetable peeler or chef's knife, remove squash skin and fibrous threads just below skin (squash should be completely orange with no white flesh). Halve squash along the length and scrape out seeds.

3. Place squash cut side down on slicing board and slice crosswise into 1/2-inch-thick pieces.

4. Toss squash with 2 tablespoons oil, 1/2 teaspoon salt, and 1/2 teaspoon pepper and lay out on rimmed baking sheet in one layer.

5. Roast squash until sides touching sheet toward back of oven are well browned, about half an hour. Rotate sheet and continue to roast until sides touching sheet toward back of oven are well browned, 6 to 10 minutes.

6. Use metal spatula to flip each piece and continue to roast until squash is very soft and sides touching sheet become browned, 10 to fifteen minutes.

7. Move squash to serving platter. Beat tahini, lemon juice, honey, remaining 1 tablespoon oil, and pinch salt together in a container.

8. Sprinkle squash with tahini dressing and drizzle with feta, pistachios, and mint.

9. Serve.

Grilled Portobello

Serves 5 pax

Ingredients

- 6 tablespoons extra-virgin olive oil
- 8 shallots
- 1 teaspoon salt
- 1 teaspoon rosemary
- 2 teaspoons lemon juice
- 6 portobello mushroom
- 1 garlic clove
- 1 teaspoon Dijon mustard
- 1 teaspoon pepper

Procedure

1. Beat 2 tablespoons oil, garlic, lemon juice, mustard, rosemary, and 1/4 teaspoon salt together in a small-sized container.

2. Sprinkle with salt and pepper to taste. Set aside for serving.

3. Thread shallots through roots and stem ends onto two 12-inch metal skewers. Use a paring knife to cut 1/2-inch crosshatch pattern, 1/4 inch deep, on tops of mushroom caps.

4. Brush shallots and mushroom caps with remaining 1/4 cup oil and sprinkle with salt and pepper.

5. Open bottom vent fully. Light large chimney starter half filled with charcoal briquettes (3 quarts).

6. When top coals are partially covered with ash, pour uniformly over grill. Set cooking grate in place, cover, and open lid vent fully.

7. Heat grill until hot, approximately five minutes.

8. Turn all burners to high, cover, and heat grill until hot, about fifteen minutes. Turn all burners to medium.

9. Clean and oil cooking grate. Place shallots and mushrooms, gill side up, on grill.

10. Cook (covered if using gas) until mushrooms have released their liquid and vegetables are charred on first side, approximately eight minutes.

11. Flip mushrooms and shallots and carry on cooking (covered if using gas) until vegetables are soft and charred on second side, approximately eight minutes. Move vegetables to serving platter.

12. Remove skewers from shallots and discard any charred outer layers.

13. Beat vinaigrette to recombine and drizzle over vegetables.

14. Serve.

Curry Lentil Dip

Serves 1 cup

Ingredients

- 2 cups water
- 1 onion
- 4 cloves garlic
- 1 cup lentils
- 2 tablespoons lemon juice
- 1 teaspoon cumin
- 1 teaspoon curry
- 1 teaspoon salt
- 2 tablespoons olive oil
- 2 tablespoons tahini

Procedure

1. Add water, onions, garlic, cumin, curry, sea salt, olive oil, and lentils to the Termoblender. Close the lid and seal.
2. Cook on high pressure for 9 minutes.
3. When it is done, quick release.
4. Open and add lemon juice, tahini. Blend with an immersion blender or food processor until smooth.
5. Add more lemon juice, olive oil, and sea salt to taste and desired consistency.
6. Serve.

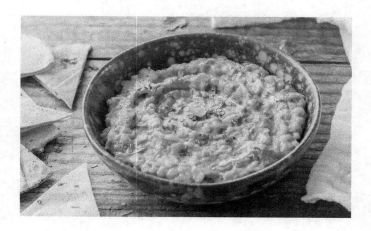

Seitan Spiced Dumplings

Serves 12 Dumplings

Ingredients

- 1 teaspoon olive oil
- 1/2 pound seitan
- 1 teaspoon ginger
- 2 onions
- 2 tablespoons tamari aminos
- 1/4 cup red wine
- 1/2 teaspoon cinnamon
- 1/4 teaspoon nutmeg
- A pinch of black pepper
- 1 teaspoon salt
- 1 teaspoon tapioca starch
- 1 tablespoon water
- 12 dumpling wrappers

Procedure

1. On sautèe setting, heat olive oil and cook seitan, ginger, and onions for 2 minutes.
2. Add tamari or coconut aminos, red win, cinnamon, nutmeg, pepper, and sea salt. Cook for a few minutes until liquid is reduced by half.
3. Add tapioca or cornstarch and cook until thickened.
4. Remove the liner from the Termoblender and set aside.
5. Lightly coat the vegetable steamer with oil.
6. Make a small bowl of water and begin to lay out a wrapper on a flat surface.
7. Spread water around the edge of the wrapper with fingertip. Add 1-2 tablespoons of filling in the middle and fold the wrapper in half, matching the edges. Place in steamer with edge sides up.
8. Repeat for all wrappers.
9. Add 1 1/2 cups of water to the Termoblender and place the steamer inside.
10. Close the lid and seal. Set to 7 minutes.
11. When it is done, quick release.
12. Serve with tamari or coconut aminos for dipping.

Fake Meat Texas Chili

Serves 6 pax

Ingredients

- 1 cup corn kernels
- 1 cup red bell pepper
- 1 teaspoon cumin
- 1 tablespoon olive oil
- 1/2 cup red onion
- 4 cloves garlic
- 1 teaspoon salt
- 1 teaspoon pepper
- 2 tablespoons chili powder
- 1 tablespoon coconut aminos
- 14 oz tomatoes
- 14 oz pinto beans
- 14 oz black beans
- 1 cup vegetable stock

Procedure

1. Heat oil in Termoblender on Sauté.
2. In the meantime, combine textured vegetable protein with stock and coconut aminos.
3. Allow to stand 4 minutes and drain.
4. Cook onions and bell peppers in heated oil for 4 minutes.
5. Add garlic and spices. Cook 1 minute.
6. Stir in remaining ingredients and lock the lid.
7. High-pressure 6 minutes.
8. Use a natural pressure release.
9. Open the lid and serve warm.

Colorful Spring Chili

Serves 4 pax

Ingredients

- 6 cherry tomatoes
- 1/4 cup celery
- 1 cup tomato paste
- 1/2 cup vegetable juice
- 2 radishes
- 8 oz cannellini beans
- 1/2 cup corn kernels
- 1 teaspoon chipotle powder
- 1 cup fennel bulb
- 1 cup carrots
- 1/4 cup onion
- 2 tablespoon shallots
- 2 cloves garlic
- 1 pinch rosemary
- 1 pinch cayenne

Procedure

1. Combine all ingredients, into the Termoblender, except the zucchinis, corn, and cherry tomatoes.
2. Lock the lid and high-pressure 8 minutes.
3. Use a natural pressure release, then release any remaining pressure with a quick-pressure release method.
4. Stir in reserved zucchinis, corn, and tomatoes. Lock the lid, and high-pressure 1 minute.
5. Perform a quick-pressure release and open the lid.
6. Serve warm.

Fake Chicken Chili

Serves 4 pax

Ingredients

- 70 oz. seitan
- 1 onion
- 2 cloves garlic
- 1 teaspoon oregano
- 1/2 cup vegetable juice
- 1 teaspoon salt
- 1 tablespoon olive oil
- 1 red bell pepper
- 14 oz. black beans
- 3 cups tomatoes
- 1 tablespoon cider vinegar
- 1 tablespoon chili powder
- 1 teaspoon chili flakes
- 1 teaspoon pepper
- 2 cups vegetable stock

Procedure

1. Heat oil in Termoblender on Sauté.
2. Cook bell pepper and onion for 4 minutes.
3. Add garlic and spices. Cook 30 seconds.
4. Stir in remaining ingredients and lock the lid.
5. High-pressure 6 minutes.
6. Use a quick-pressure release method.
7. Open the lid and stir gently. Adjust the seasonings.
8. Serve warm.

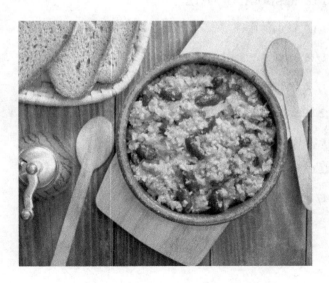

Black Bean Delight Chili

Serves 4 pax

Ingredients

- 14 oz. black beans
- 1 tablespoon chili powder
- 1 teaspoon salt
- 1 teaspoon pepper
- 1 tablespoon olive oil
- 1 red onion
- 1/2 cup carrots
- 1/2 teaspoon chili flakes
- 2 teaspoons smoked paprika
- 1 celery stalk
- 2 cups vegetable stock
- 1/4 cup cilantro

Procedure

1. Heat olive oil in Termoblender on Sauté.
2. Add onion, carrots, and celery. Cook, stirring 4 minutes.
3. Add garlic, cumin, chili powder, chili flakes, and smoked paprika.
4. Cook 30 seconds or until fragrant.
5. Add remaining ingredients and season with salt and pepper, to taste.
6. Lock the lid and High-pressure 8 minutes.
7. Use a quick pressure release method.
8. Open the lid and stir gently.
9. Serve warm.

Roasted Cauliflower

Serves 5 pax

Ingredients

- 5 slices bread
- 5 tablespoons extra-virgin olive oil
- 1 teaspoon salt
- 1/4 cup parsley
- 1 garlic clove
- 1 cauliflower
- 1 teaspoon lemon zest
- 5 lemon wedges
- 1 teaspoon pepper

Procedure

1. Trim outer leaves of cauliflower and cut stem flush with bottom of head. Turn head so stem is facing down and cut head into 3/4-inch-thick slices. Cut around core to remove florets. Discard core. Cut large florets into 11/2-inch pieces. Move florets to a container, including any small pieces that may have been created during trimming and set aside.

2. Pulse bread using a food processor to coarse crumbs, approximately ten pulses. Heat breadcrumbs, 1 tablespoon oil, pinch salt, and pinch pepper in 12-inch nonstick frying pan on moderate heat, stirring often, until breadcrumbs start to look golden brown, 3 to 5 minutes. Move crumbs to a container and wipe frying pan clean using paper towels.

3. Mix 2 tablespoons oil and cauliflower florets in now-empty frying pan and drizzle with 1 teaspoon salt and 1/2 teaspoon pepper. Cover frying pan and cook on moderate to high heat until florets get a golden color and edges just start to become

translucent (do not lift lid), approximately five minutes.

4. Remove lid and continue to cook, stirring every 2 minutes, until florets turn golden brown in many spots, about 12 minutes.

5. Push cauliflower to sides of skillet. Put in remaining 2 tablespoons oil, garlic, and lemon zest to center and cook, stirring using a rubber spatula, until aromatic, approximately half a minute.

6. Stir garlic mixture into cauliflower and continue to cook, stirring intermittently, until cauliflower becomes soft but still firm, approximately three minutes.

7. Remove from the heat, mix in parsley and sprinkle with salt and pepper to taste.

8. Move cauliflower to serving platter and drizzle with breadcrumbs.

9. Serve with lemon wedges.

Roasted Asparagus

Serves 6 pax

Ingredients

- 1/4 cup Parmesan cheese
- 1/2 cup kalamata olives
- 12 ounces cherry tomatoes
- 2 garlic cloves
- 4 pounds asparagus
- 2 tablespoons extra-virgin olive oil
- 2 tablespoons basil
- 2 teaspoons salt
- 2 teaspoons pepper

Procedure

1. Cook 1 tablespoon oil and garlic in 12-inch frying pan on moderate heat, stirring frequently, until garlic turns golden but not brown, approximately three minutes.

2. Put in tomatoes and olives and cook until tomatoes begin to break down, approximately three minutes. Move to a container.

3. Heat residual 1 tablespoon oil in now-empty frying pan on moderate to high heat until it starts to shimmer. Put in half of asparagus with tips pointed in 1 direction and remaining asparagus with tips pointed in opposite direction. Shake frying pan gently to help distribute spears evenly.

4. Put in 1 teaspoon water, cover, and cook until asparagus is bright green and still crisp, approximately five minutes.

5. Uncover, increase heat to high, and cook, moving spears around with tongs as required, until asparagus is thoroughly browned on 1 side and tip of paring knife inserted at base of largest spear meets little resistance, 5 to 7 minutes.
6. Sprinkle with salt and pepper to taste.
7. Move asparagus to serving platter, top with tomato mixture, and drizzle with basil and Parmesan.
8. Serve.

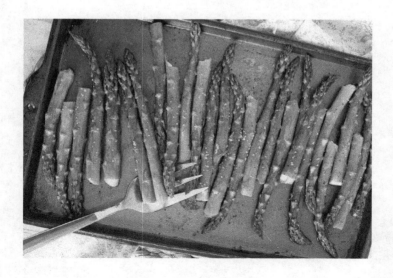

Vegetarian Recipes

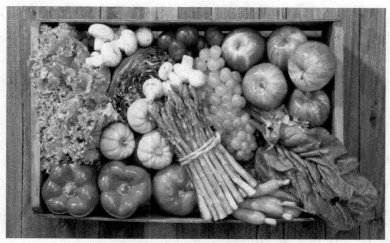

from the
Mediterranean

Vol. 2

This cookbook will boost your life right today with some fresh and new ideas! Say bye to busy meals! It's quick and easy, with these healthy and delicious recipes to feel light, lose weight and balance your nutrients supply.

Joe Madison

Guacamole

Serves 4 pax

Ingredients

- 1/3 cup red bell pepper
- Juice of 1 lime
- 2 avocados
- 1/4 teaspoon cumin
- 1 clove garlic
- 1/2 cup cilantro
- 1 jalapeño
- A pinch of red pepper flakes
- 1 teaspoon salt
- 1 teaspoon pepper
- 1 tablespoon sour cream

Procedure

1. Collect mashed avocados into a large bowl.
2. Add the rest of the ingredients and stir together.
3. Season to taste with pepper and salt.
4. Cover and chill before serving.

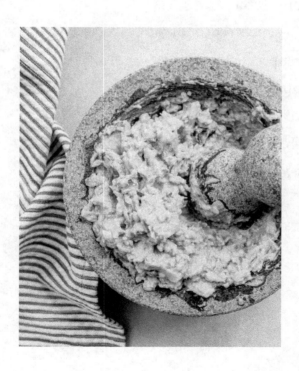

Chocolate Teff Waffles

Serves 6 pax

Ingredients

- 2 teaspoons baking powder
- 2 cups water
- 1/2 teaspoon coconut oil
- 1/3 cupcocoa powder
- 2 cups teff flour
- 1/4 cup maple syrup
- 2 tablespoons of water
- 3/4 teaspoons salt

Procedure

1. Preheat a standard size waffle iron, lightly grease if not using nonstick.
2. Collect and whisk together teff flour, cocoa powder, baking powder and salt, in a large mixing bowl, stir in the coconut oil, maple syrup, and remaining 2 cups of water.
3. Mix well by using a whisk until completely smooth.
4. Drop 1/4 cup of the batter into the waffle iron and cook for about 4 minutes per waffle.
5. Increase the time by about 1 minute if using a Belgian waffle maker.
6. Allow to cool briefly before serving.
7. Repeat for about six standard size waffles.
8. Serve hot.

Lime Bean Quinoa Salad

Serves 4 pax

Ingredients

1. 2 tablespoons brown rice syrup
2. 1 cup shredded red cabbage
3. 1/4 cup brown rice vinegar
4. Zest of 1 lime
5. Juice of 2 limes
6. 4 cups quinoa
7. 1/2 cup cilantro
8. 2 cups lima beans
9. 1 carrot
10. 1 teaspoon salt
11. 1 teaspoon black pepper

Procedure

1. Collect together brown rice vinegar, brown rice syrup, and lime zest and juice in a large bowl and whisk well to combine.
2. Add quinoa, baby lima beans, cilantro, carrot, red cabbage, salt and pepper and toss until well mixed.
3. Refrigerate before serving.

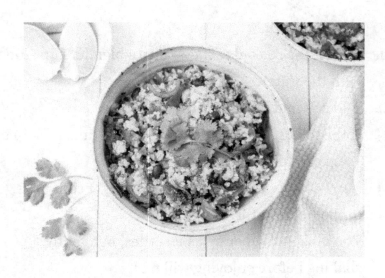

Cashew Milk

Serves 6 pax

Ingredients

- 2 cups cashews
- 1/8 teaspoon salt
- 4 cups water

Procedure

1. Collect the soaked cashews into a blender cup along with the water.
2. Add salt and blend until very smooth.
3. If the milk seems too thick for your liking, add up to 1 cup of additional water and blend.
4. Can be up to 1 week store in an airtight container, in the refrigerator.
5. The milk will separate as it settles, but gently shaking before enjoying will fix it.

Spicy Cilantro Pesto

Serves 4 pax

Ingredients

- 2 cups packed cilantro
- 1 jalapeño pepper
- 4 cloves garlic
- zest and juice of 1 lime
- 1/2 package firm tofu
- 1/2 teaspoon salt
- 1/4 cup sunflower seeds

Procedure

1. Collect jalapeño pepper, cilantro, garlic, lime zest and juice, tofu, salt, sunflower seeds in the bowl of a food processor or blender cup.
2. Blend for few minutes, until smooth and creamy.

Colcannon

Serves 4 pax

Ingredients

- 1/2 cup milk
- 2 tablespoons butter
- 11/2 tablespoons salt
- 2 pounds Yukon Gold potatoes
- 8 ounces kale
- 1/2 cup vegetable broth
- 2 tablespoons black pepper

Procedure

1. Oil your Termoblender and add the potatoes, broth and some salt.
2. Seal and cook the potatoes for 25 minutes on Stew.
3. Depressurize quickly, put inside the kale in the steamer basket, reseal and allow for the heat to wilt the kale.
4. Depressurize quickly again.
5. Mash the potatoes and stir everything together until well mixed.

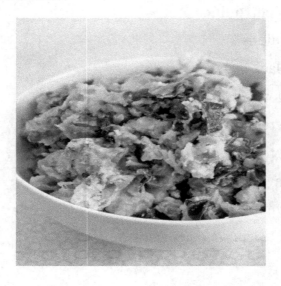

Beans with Quinoa and Corn

Serves 4 pax

Ingredients

- 1/2 cups vegetable stock
- 1 teaspoon olive oil
- 4 black pepper
- 1 cup corn kernels
- 3/4 cup quinoa
- 4 onions
- 2 black beans
- 2 cloves garlic
- 1/2 teaspoon sea salt
- 1/4 teaspoon paprika
- 1 bay leaf
- 1/2 cup cilantro
- 1/2 teaspoon black pepper

Procedure

1. Heat olive oil in a large skillet over medium heat, add green onion, garlic.
2. Cook for about 7 minutes or until tender.
3. Stir in quinoa and then add vegetable stock.
4. Season with black pepper, paprika peppercorns and salt, stir add bay leaf and allow mixture to a boil.
5. Cover and reduce the heat to simmer.
6. Keep cooking for another 20 minutes or until quinoa is soft and liquid is absorbed.
7. Stir corn kernels in the skillet, and simmer until heated through.
8. Add beans and cilantro and gently stir well to combine ingredients.
9. Serve.

Slow Fennel

Serves 6 pax

Ingredients

- 1/4 cup water
- 1/2 cup dry white wine
- 1/2 teaspoon grated lemon zest
- 2 teaspoons lemon juice
- 1 radicchio
- 2 tablespoons pine nuts
- 2 teaspoons honey
- 2 fennel bulbs
- 2 tablespoons fronds
- 3 tablespoons extra-virgin olive oil
- 1 teaspoon salt
- 1 teaspoon pepper
- 1 cup Parmesan cheese

Procedure

1. Heat oil in 12-inch frying pan on moderate heat until it starts to shimmer. Put in fennel pieces, lemon zest, 1/2 teaspoon salt, and 1/4 teaspoon pepper, then pour wine over fennel.

2. Cover, decrease the heat to moderate to low, and cook until fennel is just tender, approximately twenty minutes.

3. Increase heat to medium, flip fennel pieces, and continue to cook, uncovered, until fennel is thoroughly browned on first side and liquid is almost completely evaporated, five to ten minutes.

4. Flip fennel pieces and carry on cooking until thoroughly browned on second side, 2 to 4 minutes. Move fennel to serving platter and tent loosely with aluminium foil.

5. Put in radicchio, water, honey, and pinch salt to now-empty frying pan and cook on low heat, scraping up any browned bits, until wilted, 3 to 5 minutes.

6. Remove from the heat, mix in lemon juice and sprinkle with salt and pepper to taste.

7. Arrange radicchio over fennel and drizzle with pine nuts, minced fennel fronds, and shaved Parmesan.

Roasted Red Pepper Sauce

Serves 2 pax

Ingredients

- 2 tablespoons dill
- 1 package firm tofu
- 1/2 teaspoon black pepper
- 3 cloves garlic
- 1 lemon zest
- 1 red bell peppers
- 1 teaspoon salt

Procedure

1. Collect all ingredients in the bowl of a food processor or blender cup.
2. Blend until smooth and creamy.
3. Transfer into refrigerator in an airtight container until ready to use.

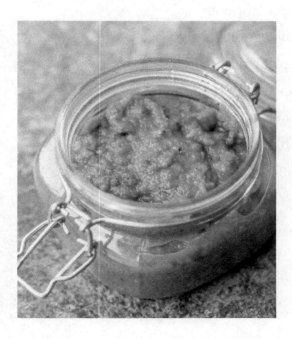

Fruited Millet Salad

Serves 4 pax

Ingredients

1. 1 cup millet
2. Zest and juice of 1 orange
3. Juice of 1 lemon
4. 1/2 cup apricots
5. 2 tablespoons brown rice syrup
6. 1 cup currants
7. 1 cup golden raisins
8. 4 apple
9. 2 tablespoons mint

Procedure

1. Allow 2 quarts of lightly salted water to a boil over high heat and add the millet.
2. Return to a boil, reduce heat to medium, cover, and keep cooking for another 14 minutes.
3. Drain from water, rinse it until millet is cool, then set aside.
4. Collect together brown rice syrup, orange juice and zest, lemon juice in a large bowl.
5. Whisk well to combine.
6. Add apple, apricots, raisins, currants, and mint stir well to mix.
7. Add the cooked millet and toss to coat.
8. Refrigerate before serving.

Bulgur, Cucumber and Tomato Salad

Serves 4 pax

Ingredients

- 2 cups bulgur
- 2 tablespoons red wine vinegar
- 1/4 cup tarragon
- 1 cup cherry tomatoes
- 1 cucumber
- 4 onions
- Zest and juice of 2 lemons
- 3 cloves garlic
- 1 teaspoon red pepper flakes
- 1 teaspoon salt
- 1 teaspoon black pepper

Procedure

1. Collect 3 cups water into a medium size pot, place over medium high heat, allow to boil, then add bulgur.
2. Remove pot from the heat, cover with a tight fitting lid, and allow it to sit, for about 15 minutes or until the water is absorbed and the bulgur is tender.
3. Spread the bulgur on a baking sheet and allow to cool at room temperature.
4. Transfer the cooled bulgur to a bowl, add all the remaining ingredients, and mix well to combine.
5. Chill for 1 hour before serving.

Buttery Tofu Tomatoes

Serves 6 pax

Ingredients

- 1/8 teaspoon turmeric
- 4 cloves garlic
- 1 1/2 tablespoons garam masala
- 2 tablespoons olive oil
- 1 onion
- 2 tablespoons ginger
- 2 teaspoons cumin
- 1/4 cup water
- 15 ounces tofu
- 28 ounces tomatoes
- 3 tablespoons butter
- 1/4 cup milk
- Brown basmati rice, for serving

Procedure

1. Heat the olive oil on the sauté setting and cook the onion for 5 minutes. Add the garlic and cook one more minute.

2. Add the tofu, water, ginger, tomatoes, cumin, garam masala, turmeric, and salt in the Termoblender, seal the lid, and cook on high 4 minutes.

3. Remove the lid and stir in the nondairy milk and butter until melted. Serve over rice.

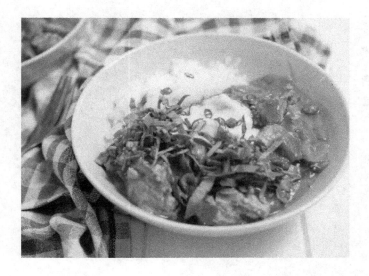

Wheat Berry Salad

Serves 4 pax

Ingredients

- 2 cups berries
- 1 cup rice syrup
- 1/2 cup cranberries
- 2 celery stalks
- 2 tablespoons tarragon
- 1 cup onion
- 1 cup apple vinegar
- 1 bosc pear
- 1 teaspoon salt
- 1 teaspoon black pepper

Procedure

1. Collect 5 cups water in to a medium size saucepan, place over medium high heat then allow to boil, add wheat berries. Keep cooking over high heat.
2. Reduce heat to medium, low heat cover and keep cooking for about about 13/4 hours or until the wheat berries are tender.
3. Drain the excess water from the pan and rinse the berries until cool.
4. Collect all the other ingredients together in a large bowl.
5. Add the cooled wheat berries and mix together. Make is well.
6. Chill for 1 hour before serving.

Quinoa, Black Bean and Corn Salad

Serves 4 pax

Ingredients

- 1 red bell pepper
- 1 tablespoon cumin seeds
- 2 cups quinoa
- 1 tablespoon cumin seeds
- 4 ears corn
- 1/2 red onion
- Zest of 1 lime
- Juice of 2 limes
- 3 cups black beans
- 6 onions
- 1 cup cilantro
- 1 jalapeño
- 1 teaspoon salt

Procedure

1. Collect all ingredients together in a large bowl and mix well.

2. Transfer to refrigerator and chill for 1 hour before serving.

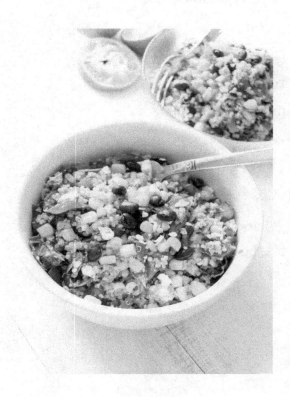

Potato, Corn and Bean Soup

Serves 8 pax

Ingredients

- 8 cups vegetable stock
- 1 onion
- 1 tablespoon thyme
- 7 red skin potatoes
- 1 pound green beans
- 6 ears corn
- 2 cloves garlic
- 3 cups cooked navy beans
- 1 teaspoon salt
- 1 teaspoon black pepper

Procedure

1. Sauté onion in a large pot over medium heat for about 10 minutes, add water 1 tablespoons at a time to keep them from sticking to the pot, add garlic and thyme.
2. Keep cooking for another 1 minute, add vegetable stock, green beans, potatoes, and corn, cover and keep cooking over medium heat, for about 15 minutes.
3. Add navy beans, season with salt and pepper, cook for another 10 minutes or until the vegetables are tender.

Bean Soup, Rosemary and Lemon

Serves 6 pax

Ingredients

- 6 cups vegetable stock
- 2 teaspoons rosemary
- 2 celery stalk
- 2 leeks
- Zest of 2 lemons
- 2 cloves garlic
- 6 potatoes
- 2 cups beans
- 1 teaspoon salt
- 1 teaspoon black pepper

Procedure

1. Collect leeks and celery in a large pot, sauté over medium high heat for about 10 minutes, add water 1 tablespoons at a time to keep the vegetables from sticking to the pot.

2. Add garlic, rosemary and keep cooking for another 1 minute, add potatoes, beans, and vegetable stock. Allow to boil over medium high heat.

3. Reduce heat to medium low heat, then cover and keeping cooking for 20 minutes more or until the potatoes are tender.

4. Add lemon zest, season with pepper and salt. Further cook for another 5 minutes.

5. Serve.

Tomatoes and Red Pepper Soup

Serves 4 pax

Ingredients

- 3 tomatoes
- 2 onions
- 1 teaspoon thyme
- 2 red bell peppers
- 1/4 cup basil
- 2 cloves garlic
- 1 teaspoon salt
- 1 teaspoon black pepper

Procedure

1. Collect red pepper and onions in a large saucepan, sauté over medium high heat for about 10 minutes.
2. Add water 1 tablespoons at a time to keep the vegetables from sticking to the pot, add garlic, thyme.
3. Keep cooking for another 1 minute, add tomatoes, cover and cook for 20 minutes more.
4. Transfer soup in to immersion blender cup or in batches in a blender cup with a tight fitting lid, covered with a towel, Puree the soup.
5. Return the soup to the pot and season with pepper and salt.
6. Serve and garnished with the basil.

Soy Chorizo & Black Bean Stew

Serves 4 pax

Ingredients

- 1 tablespoon olive oil
- 1 shallot
- 2 tablespoons vegan bouillon
- 2 oz black beans
- 6 oz soy chorizo
- 1/2 bell pepper
- 1/4 teaspoon pepper
- 1/8 teaspoon cayenne pepper
- Zest of 1 lime
- 1/4 teaspoon cumin
- 1/4 teaspoon chipotle chili powder
- 1/4 teaspoon salt

Procedure

1. Use the sauté setting to cook the shallot for 5 minutes, then add the garlic and bell pepper.
2. Cook an additional 3 minutes before adding the rest of the ingredients to the Termoblender.
3. Seal the lid and cook on high 6 minutes.
4. Serve in bowls topped with vegan sour cream and tortilla chips.

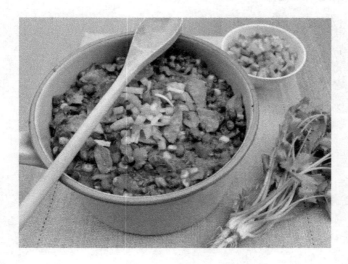

Homemade Vegetable Stock

Ingredients

- 4 green onions
- 1/4 teaspoon salt
- 1 cup hemp milk
- 1 cucumber
- 1/4 teaspoon black pepper
- 1/4 cup cilantro
- Juice of 1/2 lime
- 2 avocados

Procedure

1. Heat a large stockpot over medium high heat, add in olive oil. Heat until hot, add onion, potatoes, carrots, and yam and keep cooking for another 4 – 5 minutes.
2. Add spinach and garlic, and cook for 3 minutes. Add water, parsley, bay leaves, pepper, tomatoes, salt and any other herbs you like.
3. Reduce heat to low. Simmer for a few hours, or longer.
4. Collect mixture in a blender or food processor, blend until completely smooth, and use as a stock (you will need to add more water to it) or strain out and discard all the vegetables and use the remaining stock for soups, stews, and risottos.

Roasted Tomato Soup

Serves 6 pax

Ingredients

- 32 ounces vegetable stock
- 2 carrots
- 1 teaspoon black pepper
- 1 red bell pepper
- 1 tablespoon olive oil
- 1 onion
- 5 cloves garlic
- 1 teaspoon salt
- 6 tomatoes
- 1/4 cup basil

Procedure

1. Preheat the oven to 400°F. Lay tomatoes and garlic on a large, lightly oiled cookie sheet.
2. Sprinkle with pepper and salt and roast for about 45 – 50 minutes or until soft. Allow to cool, then remove the skin of the tomatoes.
3. While, waiting, add 1 tablespoon olive oil in a small saucepan, place over medium heat, add onions and cook for about 3 minutes or until onions begin to soften, add bell pepper and keep cooking until peppers are soft.
4. Reduce heat. Simmer carrots in a 2 q uart stockpot, in the vegetable stock. Add the cooked onions and peppers, the tomatoes and garlic after they have roasted. Allow to a boil, add basil. Simmer for about 5 – 10 minutes.
5. Remove from heat, pour mixture in a food processor or blender, blend until smooth.
6. If the mixture is too thick, add water to thin it.
7. Return the soup to the stockpot, adjust season to taste, and heat through.

Fava Beans and Vegetable Soup

Serves 4 pax

Ingredients

- 1/2 cup white wine
- 2 cups fava beans
- 1/2 cup carrots
- 2 leeks
- 1 cup green beans
- 1 cup asparagus
- 32 ounces organic vegetable stock
- 3/4 cup basil
- 1 tablespoon olive oil
- 3 cloves garlic
- 1 teaspoon black pepper
- 1 teaspoon salt

Procedure

1. Heat oil over In a large stockpot, over medium high heat and add the leeks, cook for about 3 minutes or until leek become soft.
2. Add carrots, asparagus, fava beans keep cooking for another 4 – 5 minutes.
3. Add cooked green beans and garlic, and cook for a minute, add vegetable stock, wine, and basil.
4. Reduce heat to low. Simmer until the beans are cooked, and the flavors have blended.
5. Adjust season to taste. Garnish with parsley.

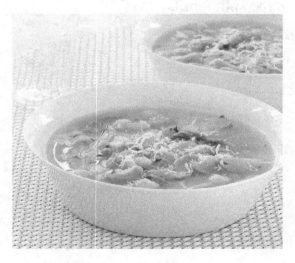

Carrot and Lentil Soup

Serves 4 pax

Ingredients

- 2 tablespoons olive oil
- 1 teaspoon paprika
- 1 celery stick
- 2 teaspoons cumin
- 1 onion
- 1 teaspoon coriander
- 1 teaspoon cilantro
- 1 cup red split lentils
- 1 potato
- 6 carrots
- 1 teaspoon salt
- 1 teaspoon black pepper
- 2 bay leaves

Procedure

1. Heat oil in a large, heavy saucepan over medium low heat, add onion cook for 3 minutes, stirring occasionally, add carrots, celery and potato, cook for about 5 minutes, stirring occasionally. Stir in the paprika, ground coriander, cumin and chili powder, if using. Keep cooking for another 1 minute.

2. Stir in the lentils, stock, and bay leaves. Allow to boil, then reduce the heat and simmer, half covered, over low heat, stirring occasionally to prevent the lentils from sticking to the bottom of the saucepan. Cook for 25 minutes, or until the lentils are tender.

3. Remove and discard the bay leaves. Transfer to a food processor or blender, or use a handheld immersion blender, and process the soup until smooth.

4. Return to the saucepan and reheat. Season with pepper and salt, add extra chili powder, if desired. Ladle into warm bowls and garnish with cilantro before serving.

Coconut and Mango Quinoa

Serves 4 pax

Ingredients

- 2 cup white quinoa
- 1/4 cup coconut chips
- 1 mango
- 2 cups coconut milk
- 1 inch ginger
- 2/3 cup blueberries
- 1/3 cup sugar
- Juice of 1 lime
- 4 lime wedges

Procedure

1. Collect coconut milk and quinoa into a small saucepan. Place over medium high heat and allow to boil. Reduce the heat, cover, and simmer for 20 minutes or until most of the liquid has evaporated.
2. Remove from heat, but leave the pan covered for an additional 10 minutes to allow the grains to swell. Fluff up with a fork, transfer to a bowl, cool.
3. Meanwhile, peel the mango, discard the pit, and coarsely chop the flesh (you will need 2 cups). Put the mango into a food processor with the sugar and lime juice. Squeeze ginger in a garlic press and add the juice to the mango mixture. Process for 30 seconds to make a smooth puree.
4. Mix the mango mixture into the cooled quinoa and allow to stand for 30 minutes.
5. Divide the mixture among four bowls and sprinkle with the blueberries and coconut chips. Decorate with lime wedges and serve.

Marinated Olives

Serves 8 pax

Ingredients

- 1 cup black olives
- 2 teaspoons lemon zest
- 2 teaspoons oregano
- 2 teaspoons thyme
- 1 garlic clove
- 1 shallot
- 1/2 teaspoon red pepper flakes
- 1/2 teaspoon salt
- 3/4 cup extra-virgin olive oil

Procedure

1. Wash olives comprehensively, then drain and pat dry using paper towels.
2. Toss olives with the rest of the ingredients in a container, cover, put inside your fridge for minimum 4 hours or for maximum 4 days.
3. Allow to sit at room temperature for minimum half an hour before you serve.

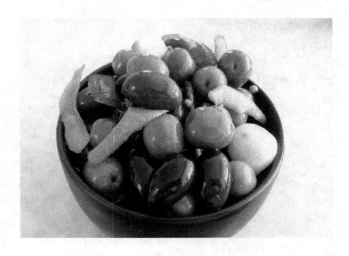

Saffroned Caulipeas

Serves 8 pax

Ingredients

- 11/2 teaspoons sugar
- 2 tablespoons sherry vinegar
- 5 garlic cloves
- 1/2 cauliflower
- 1/2 lemon
- 1 cup chickpeas
- 1 sprig rosemary
- 1/8 teaspoon saffron threads
- 1/3 cup extra-virgin olive oil
- 2 teaspoons smoked paprika

Procedure

1. Bring 2 quarts water to boil in a big saucepan. Put in cauliflower and 1 tablespoon salt and cook until florets start to become tender, approximately three minutes. Drain florets and move to paper towel–lined baking sheet.

2. Mix 1/4 cup hot water and saffron in a container; set aside. Heat oil and garlic in small saucepan over moderate to low heat until aromatic and starting to sizzle but not brown, four to eight minutes. Mix in sugar, paprika, and rosemary and cook until aromatic, approximately half a minute.

3. Remove from the heat, mix in saffron mixture, vinegar, salt and pepper.

4. Mix florets, saffron mixture, chickpeas, and lemon in a big container. Cover and place in the fridge, stirring intermittently, for minimum 4 hours or for maximum 3 days.

5. To serve, discard rosemary sprig, move cauliflower and chickpeas to serving bowl using a slotted spoon, and drizzle with parsley.

Not So Fat Guacamole

Ingredients

- 1 cup edamame
- 1 lime zest
- Juice of 2 limes
- 1 teaspoon salt
- 1 red onion
- 1/4 cup cilantro
- 1 teaspoon garlic
- 1 cup broccoli
- 2 tomatoes
- A pinch of cayenne pepper

Procedure

1. Collect edamame in a medium size saucepan, add water to cover.
2. Place over medium high heat and allow to boil and cook for about 5 minutes. Drain and rinse the edamame until cooled.
3. Place broccoli in in a double boiler or steamer basket and steam for about 8 minutes, or until very tender. Drain and rinse the broccoli until cooled.
4. Collect edamame and broccoli together in a food processor or blebder cup, blend for few minutes or until smooth and creamy. Add water if need to achieve a creamy texture.
5. Transfer pureed mixture into a bowl, add lime zest and juice, cilantro, tomatoes, garlic, onion, salt, and cayenne. Stir together to mix well.
6. Transfer to refrigerator and chill until ready to serve.

Spicy Asian Quinoa Salad

Serves 6 pax

Ingredients

- 4 cups quinoa
- 3 cup rice vinegar
- 4 cups spinach
- 4 cloves garlic
- Zest and juice of 2 limes
- 2 teaspoons red pepper flakes
- 2 tablespoons ginger
- 2 cups adzuki beans,
- 3/4 cup bean sprouts
- 1/2 cup cilantro
- 1 teaspoon salt
- 6 onions

Procedure

1. Collect together brown rice vinegar, crushed red pepper flakes, lime zest and juice, garlic and ginger in a large bowl, mix well.
2. Add quinoa, mung bean sprouts adzuki beans,, green onions, cilantro and salt and toss to coat.

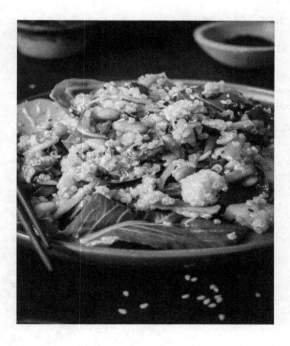

Rice Salad with Fennel, Orange and Chickpeas

Serves 4 pax

Ingredients

- 2 cups basmati rice
- 1 orange
- 2 cups chickpeas
- 1 cup parsley
- 1 cup white wine vinegar
- 1 fennel bulb
- 1/2 teaspoon red pepper flakes

Procedure

1. Rinse rice under cold running water and drain. Transfer to a medium size pot with 3 cups of cold water.
2. Place over medium high heat, allow to to boil. Reduce heat to medium, low heat cover and cook for about 45 – 50 minutes, or until the rice is tender.
3. While rice is cooking, collect white wine vinegar, chickpeas, crushed red pepper flakes, fennel, orange zest and segments, and parsley together in a large bowl and mix together, make sure is well mixed.
4. Once rice is cooked, add the rice to the bowl and mix together.
5. Serve.

Quinoa Arugula Salad

Serves 4 pax

Ingredients

- 1 red bell pepper
- 2 cup brown rice vinegar
- 4 cups arugula
- 2 tablespoons pine nuts
- 1 teaspoon pepper
- 2 cups quinoa
- 2 oranges zest and juice
- 1 lime zest and juice
- 1 red onion
- 1 teaspoon salt

Procedure

1. Rinse quinoa under cold running water and drain. Collect 3 cups of water in a medium size pot, place over medium heat and allow to boil. Add quinoa and allow to boil again over medium high heat.
2. Reduce heat to medium, low heat cover, and keep cooking for about 15 – 20 minutes, or until the quinoa is tender.
3. Drain any excess water, spread the quinoa on a baking sheet, and refrigerate until cool.
4. While quinoa is cooling, collect orange zest and juice, lime zest and juice, arugula, brown rice vinegar, red pepper, onion, pine nuts, and salt and pepper together in a large bowl.
5. Add the cooled quinoa and chill for an hour before serving.

Sweet Potatoes Chickpeas Biryani

Serves 6 pax

Ingredients

- 2 tablespoons vegan bouillon
- 1/4 teaspoon salt
- 1/4 teaspoon pepper
- 2 cups water
- 1 onion
- 2 tablespoons olive oil
- 1 teaspoon turmeric
- 2 teaspoons garam masala
- 1 sweet potato
- 15 ounces chickpeas
- 8 ounces cauliflower
- 1 bell pepper
- 1 teaspoon ginger
- 6 cups cooked rice

Procedure

1. Heat the olive oil on the sauté setting and cook the onion for 5 minutes.
2. Add the bell pepper and cook for 2 more minutes before adding the rest of the ingredients.
3. Seal the lid and cook on high 4 minutes.
4. Serve on top of rice.

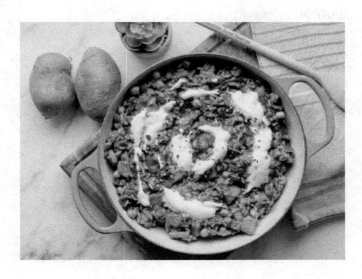

Edamame, Potatoes, Chard

Serves 4 pax

Ingredients

- 2 tablespoons lemon juice
- 2 teaspoons olive oil
- 1 teaspoon salt
- pounds potatoes
- 1 onion
- 3 garlic cloves
- 1/2 cup dry white wine
- 1/4 teaspoon black pepper
- 8 ounces Swiss chard
- 3 cups edamame
- 1/2 cup vegetable broth

Procedure

1. Warm the oil in your Termoblender.
2. Add the onion and soften for 5 minutes.
3. Add the wine, garlic and simmer 2 minutes.
4. Add the edamame, potatoes and broth. Salt and pepper a bit.
5. Seal and cook on Stew for 30 minutes. Release the pressure quickly.
6. Put the chard in the steamer basket and lower on top of the rest. Seal and Steam for 2 minutes.
7. Release the pressure quickly and serve.

Vegan Scramble

Serves 4 pax

Ingredients

- 12 pcs asparagus
- 1/2 tsp pepper
- 7 oz tofu
- 1/2 cup tomatoes
- 4 slices vegan bread
- 1/4 tsp turmeric
- 1/2 tsp salt

Procedure

1. Place the dried tomatoes in a bowl and pour over hot water. Allow to sit until the tomatoes are soft.
2. Meanwhile, cut the tofu and crumble into smaller pieces. Pour about 1/4 cup water into a frying pan heated over medium-high temperature.
3. Add the crumbled tofu, turmeric and season with salt and pepper. Cover the pan and cook for 8-10 minutes, or until the tofu is cooked.
4. Top the bread slices with the cooked tofu scramble, asparagus, and dried tomatoes.
5. Season with salt and pepper before serving.

Spelt and Beans Burritos

Ingredients

- 1 teaspoon chili powder
- 1 teaspoons grapeseed oil
- 1 bell pepper
- 3/4 cup onion
- 1 teaspoon paprika
- 1 teaspoon cumin
- 1/2 teaspoon turmeric
- 1 cup spelt berries
- 1 tablespoon cashew sauce
- 6 tablespoons cilantro
- 1 jalapeño pepper
- 6x8 inch vegan tortillas
- 2 oz black beans
- 1/2 teaspoon salt

Procedure

1. Preheat oven to 400°F.
2. Collect oil, onion, garlic, peppers, turmeric, paprika, chili powder, cumin and salt in a large skillet.
3. Cook for about 6 minutes over medium high heat, stirring frequently, until the peppers and onion just soften while remaining slightly crisp.
4. Stir spelt and beans into the mixture, cook for another 4 minutes, add sauce.
5. Reduce heat to simmer and cook for another 2 minutes or until thickened and fragrant.
6. Divide mixture among the flour tortillas (1/2 cup per tortilla), top with 1 tablespoon cilantro, and roll burrito style.
7. Lightly coat each burrito with cooking spray.
8. Bake for about 15 minutes or until light golden brown.
9. Serve immediately with extra cheesy sauce and hot sauce.

Spicy Orange and Black Beans Stew

Serves 6 pax

Ingredients

- 14 ounces tomatoes
- 1 teaspoon smoked paprika
- 14 ounces black beans
- 1 teaspoon chipotle chili powder
- 1 teaspoon hot sauce
- 1/8 teaspoon cayenne pepper
- 1 teaspoon liquid smoke
- 1 tablespoon cilantro
- Juice of 1 lime
- Juice of 1 orange
- 2 cloves garlic
- 1 tablespoon jerk seasoning
- 18 crispy tortilla strips

Procedure

1. Combine everything but the cilantro and tortilla strips in the Termoblender, seal the lid, and cook on high for 6 minutes.
2. You can leave the soup chunky or puree it with an immersion blender until smooth.
3. Top with chopped cilantro and tortilla strips.

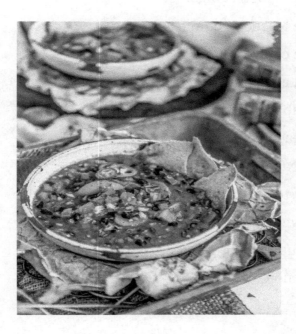

Artichokes and Eggplants

Serves 6 pax

Ingredients

- 1/2 cup kalamata olives
- 1 red bell pepper
- 2 teaspoons ginger
- 1/2 teaspoon cumin
- 1/2 cup vegetable broth
- 1/4 cup parsley
- 1 tablespoon lemon juice
- 1 teaspoon lemon zest
- 2 teaspoons olive oil
- 1/4 teaspoon salt
- 1 eggplant
- 2 cups artichoke hearts
- 1 onion

Procedure

1. Warm the oil in your Termoblender.
2. Add the onion and soften for 5 minutes.
3. Add the ginger and cook another minute.
4. Add the eggplant and cook for 5 minutes with the lid still off.
5. Add the spices and stir well.
6. Add the remaining ingredients and stir well again.
7. Seal and cook on Stew for 35 minutes.
8. Depressurize naturally and serve over couscous.

Ratatouille

Serves 6 pax

Ingredients

- 1 bell pepper
- 6 tomatoes
- 1/2 teaspoon marjoram
- 1/2 teaspoon basil
- 2 teaspoons salt
- 2 teaspoons black pepper
- 1 onion
- 3 garlic cloves
- 1 eggplant
- 4 zucchini
- 1/4 cup basil
- 2 teaspoons olive oil

Procedure

1. Warm the oil in your Termoblender.
2. Soften the onion for 5 minutes.
3. Add the garlic, dry basil, and marjoram for a minute.
4. Add the remaining ingredients except for the fresh basil.
5. Seal and cook for 25 minutes on Stew.
6. Depressurize quickly and stir in the fresh basil.

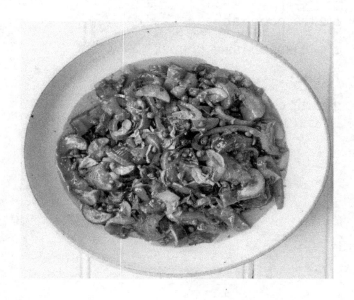

Green Beans Casserole

Serves 4 pax

Ingredients

- 8 ounces cream cheese
- 6 ounces fried onions
- 3/4 cup vegetable broth
- 2 pounds green beans
- 2 teaspoons olive oil
- 1/2 teaspoon salt
- 1/4 teaspoon black pepper
- 1 onion
- 2 garlic cloves

Procedure

1. Warm the oil in your Termoblender.
2. Add the onion and soften for 5 minutes.
3. Add the garlic and cook another minute.
4. Put the onion in a blender and blend with cream cheese, broth, salt and pepper.
5. Mix the green beans, mushrooms, and onion mix in the Termoblender.
6. Seal and cook on Stew for 25 minutes.
7. Depressurize quickly and stir some of the onions in, sprinkling the rest on top.

Potatoes Tapenade

Serves 5 pax

Ingredients

- 2 pounds Yukon Gold potatoes
- 9 ounces artichoke hearts
- 1/2 cup pitted green olives
- 1/4 cup sun-dried tomatoes
- 1 onion
- 3 garlic cloves
- 2 tablespoons capers
- 2 teaspoons olive oil
- 1/2 teaspoon basil
- 1/2 teaspoon thyme
- 2 teaspoons salt
- 2 teaspoons black pepper

Procedure

1. Blend the artichokes, olives, tomatoes, and capers into a fine mince.
2. Warm the oil in your Termoblender.
3. Soften the onion in the hot oil for 5 minutes.
4. Stir in the basil, garlic, and thyme and cook another minute. Remove.
5. Layer the potatoes at the bottom of your Termoblender.
6. Top with half the onions, then half the blend.
7. Repeat the three layers.
8. Seal and cook on Meat for 35 minutes.

Chimichurri Squash

Serves 4 pax

Ingredients

- 3 oz spaghetti squash
- 2 cups water
- 1 bunch of parsley
- 4 garlic cloves
- 1/4 cup olive oil
- 2 teaspoons oregano
- 3/4 teaspoon salt
- 1/2 teaspoon black pepper
- 1/4 teaspoon red pepper flakes
- 2 tablespoons red wine vinegar
- A pinch of sugar

Procedure

1. Pierce the squash all over with a fork.
2. Put it in your Termoblender with the water and seal.
3. Cook on Stew for 65 minutes.
4. Blend the garlic, oregano, parsley, salt, black pepper, red pepper, and sugar into a paste.
5. Add the vinegar and oil and blend until smooth.
6. When the squash has cooked, depressurize the Termoblender naturally.
7. Remove the squash and shred, then stir in the sauce.

Vegetables with Beans and Barley

Serves 4 pax

Ingredients

- 1/2 cup green peas
- 1/2 cup pearl barley
- 1/4 cup sage
- 1 carrot
- 1 fennel bulb
- 2 garlic cloves
- 2 teaspoons olive oil
- 1 onion
- cups cannellini beans
- 1 cup cherry tomatoes
- 1 cup vegetable broth
- 1 red bell pepper
- 1 zucchini

Procedure

1. Warm the oil in your Termoblender.
2. Add the onion and soften 5 minutes.
3. Add the garlic and cook another minute.
4. Add the carrot, celery, bell pepper, fennel, zucchini, barley, beans, and broth.
5. Seal and cook on Stew for 12 minutes.
6. Release the pressure and add the tomatoes and peas.
7. Seal and cook on Stew for 5 more minutes.
8. Release the pressure naturally.

Quinoa Tabbouleh

Serves 4 pax

Ingredients

- 2 cups quinoa
- 1 cucumber
- Zest of 1 lemon
- Juice of 2 lemons
- 4 roma tomatoes
- 2 cups chickpeas
- 1 cup parsley
- 8 onions
- 2 tablespoons mint
- 1 teaspoon salt
- 1 teaspoon black pepper

Procedure

1. Collect all ingredients together in a large bowl.
2. Transfer to refrigerator and chill for 1 hour before serving.

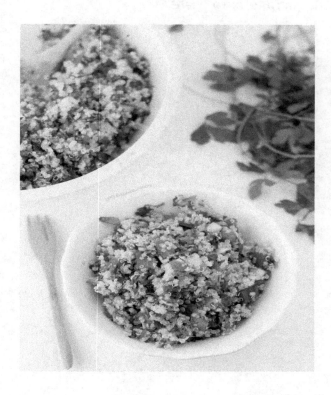

Eggplant Stew

Serves 5 pax

Ingredients

- 2 bell peppers
- 1/4 cup tomato paste
- 1 bunch parsley
- 3 tomatoes
- 1 tsp salt
- 2 tsp sugar
- 2 oz almonds
- 4 eggplants

Procedure

1. Plug in your Termoblender and grease the bottom of a stainless steel insert with two tablespoons of olive oil.
2. Make the first layer with halved eggplants tucking the ends gently to fit in.
3. Now, make the second layer with finely chopped tomatoes and red bell peppers. Spread the tomato paste evenly over the vegetables and sprinkle with finely chopped almonds. Add the remaining olive oil, salt, and pepper.
4. Pour about 1 1/2 cup of water and close the lid. Set the release steam handle and press "Manual" button. Set the timer for 13 minutes and cook on high pressure.
5. Now, press "Cancel" button and perform a quick release. Let it chill for 10 minutes before removing the lid.

Greek Dolmades

Serves 5 pax

Ingredients

- 1/2 cup olive oil
- 3 garlic cloves
- 2 tbsp mint
- 2 tsp salt
- 40 wine leaves
- 1 cup long grain rice
- 1/4 cup lemon juice
- 2 tsp pepper

Procedure

1. Wash the leaves thoroughly, one at a time. Place on a clean working surface. Set aside.
2. In a medium-sized bowl, combine rice with three tablespoons of olive oil, garlic, mint, salt, and pepper.
3. Place one wine leaf at a time on a working surface and add rice filling at the bottom end. Fold the leaf over the filling towards the center. Bring the two sides in towards the center and roll them up tightly.
4. Plug in your Termoblender and grease the bottom of the stainless steel insert with two tablespoons of olive oil. Make a layer of wine leaves and then gently transfer previously prepared rolls.
5. Add the remaining oil, 2 cups of water, and lemon juice. Close the lid and set the steam release handle. Press "Manual" button and set the timer for 30 minutes. Cook on high pressure.
6. When done, press "Cancel" button and turn off the pot. Let it stand for 10 minutes to chill. Remove the dolmades from the pot and chill overnight in the refrigerator.

Spicy Sweet Chutney

Serves 4 cups

Ingredients

- 1/2 cup cider vinegar
- 1/3 cup raisins
- 1 cup sugar
- 2 shallots
- 2 teaspoons ginger
- 1/4 teaspoon salt
- 5 apples
- 2 cups fruit

Procedure

1. Combine all the ingredients in your Termoblender and mix well.
2. Cook on Stew for 25 minutes.
3. Release the pressure naturally.
4. Simmer with the lid off for another 5 minutes.

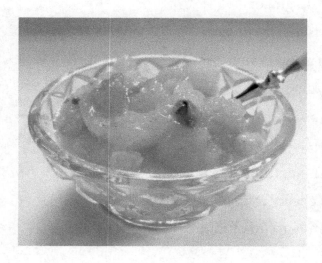

Sweet Chickpeas Stew

Serves 4 pax

Ingredients

- 1 apple
- 1/2 cup raisins
- 1/2 cup button mushrooms
- 2 carrots
- 1 cup chickpea
- 1 tsp ginger
- 1 tsp curry powder
- 1/2 cup orange juice
- 1/2 tsp salt
- 1 onion
- An handful of string beans
- An handful of peanuts
- 4 cherry tomatoes
- An handful of mint

Procedure

1. Plug in your Termoblender and combine all ingredients in the stainless steel insert. Add enough water to cover and press "Manual" button.
2. Adjust the steam release handle and set the timer for 8 minutes. Cook on high pressure.
3. When done, press "Cancel" button and release the steam naturally.
4. Let it stand for 10 minutes before opening and serving.
5. Serve.

Garlic, Kale and Beans Stew

Serves 6 pax

Ingredients

- 1 teaspoon olive oil
- 2 cloves garlic
- 1/2 teaspoon salt
- 1/2 teaspoon pepper
- 1 onion
- 1 tablespoon oregano
- 4 cups kale
- 2 oz white beans
- 4 cups water
- 1 bay leaf
- 1 tablespoon balsamic vinegar

Procedure

1. Cook the onion for 5 minutes using the sauté setting, then add the garlic, salt and pepper. Continue cooking for 1 minute before adding the balsamic vinegar.

2. Add the water, bay leaf, oregano, and beans to the onion mixture.

3. Seal the lid and cook on high 6 minutes and remove lid. Discard the bay leaf.

4. Return to sauté setting and add the chopped kale. Simmer for about 30 minutes, until the kale is tender.

Cranberry Apple Chutney

Serves 4 cups

Ingredients

- 1/2 cup cranberries
- 1/4 cup cider vinegar
- 1 teaspoon ginger
- 1 lemon zeste
- 2 shallots
- 12 ounces cranberries
- 2 cups sugar

Procedure

1. Combine all the ingredients in your Termoblender and mix well.
2. Seal and cook on Stew for 25 minutes.
3. Release the pressure naturally.
4. Simmer for another 5 minutes with the lid off to thicken.

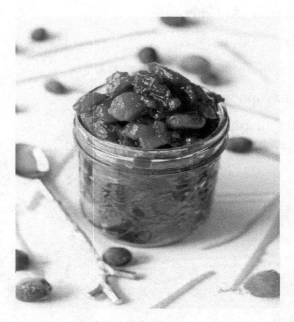

Oat, Yogurt and Berries Muffins

Ingredients

- 1/2 cup dry sweetener
- 2/3 cup milk
- 2 cup berries
- 1/2 cup soy yogurt
- 3/4 teaspoon salt
- 2 cups oat flour
- 2 teaspoons pure vanilla extract
- 1 tablespoon baking powder
- 1/2 cup applesauce

Procedure

1. Preheat oven to 350°F. Line a 12 cup muffin pan with silicone liners or have ready a nonstick or silicone muffin pan.
2. Sift together flour, baking powder, dry sweetener and salt, in a medium size mixing bowl.
3. Make a well in the center and pour in the plant based milk, yogurt, applesauce and vanilla. Stir together the wet ingredients in the well.
4. Then mix the wet and dry ingredients together just until the dry ingredients are moistened (do not overmix).
5. Fold in the berries.
6. Fill each muffin cup 3/4 of the way and transfer to oven and bake for about 22 – 26 minutes or until a knife inserted through the center should come out clean.
7. Allow muffins cool to completely, for about 20 minutes, then carefully run a knife around the edges of each muffin to remove.

Many Thanks...

To all of you who are arrived until here.
I am glad you enjoyed my recipes.
Now you stepped a little further into the vegetarian
world, so let me share one more tip with you.
The cookbooks contained in this boundle take part of a
vegetarian book series of 6 pieces, each one an
unmissable councilor of your library.
It will become essential in your practice and for your
shelves.
So, if you decide to improve your healthy-life knowledge
with my help, check out also the other books.

Joe Madison